This page was intentionally left blank

Dr. Harry Chew

ERECT CURE

A Chronicle of intimate Restoration

Dedication

In the tender folds of connection and the resilient spirit of love, this book is dedicated to every individual and partner who has confronted the challenges of erectile dysfunction (ED) with unwavering courage and an open heart.

To those who have dared to share their vulnerabilities, who have weathered the storm of intimate struggles, and who have emerged stronger, this dedication is a heartfelt tribute to your resilience.

In honoring the triumphs, setbacks, and the profound human experience, "Erect Cure" is dedicated to those who believe in the transformative power of understanding, empathy, and the boundless heights of love.

May this book serve as a companion on your journey—a beacon of hope, a source of inspiration, and a reminder that, amidst the shadows, there exists a Penile of revitalized intimacy waiting to be embraced.

With deep appreciation for the stories shared and the connections forged, this book is dedicated to you—the protagonists of your own narratives, the architects of love's triumphs, and the seekers of a lifted Penile.

— Dr. Harry Chew

Table of Contents

Preface

In the tantalizing preface of "Erect Cure," prepare to step into a narrative that transcends the conventional boundaries of conversations about erectile dysfunction (ED). This isn't just a book; it's an intimate odyssey into the realms of human connection, vulnerability, and the electrifying journey toward renewed passion.

As you flip through these pages, imagine not just words on paper but the heartbeat of shared experiences pulsating through the narrative. "Erect Cure" is a symphony of stories, an anthem of resilience, and a celebration of the intricate dance between individuals and their partners in the face of ED.

Buckle up for a rollercoaster of emotions as we navigate the labyrinth of love, embracing the nuances that make every relationship unique. This preface isn't just an introduction; it's an exhilarating overture, inviting you into a world where vulnerability is a strength, where challenges are catalysts for transformation, and where the Penile of connection awaits.

Picture this preface as the curtain rising on a stage where love takes center stage, conquering obstacles and emerging stronger. "Erect Cure" isn't your ordinary guide; it's a compass for those navigating the uncharted waters of intimate relationships affected by ED. Through tales that resonate, characters that inspire, and triumphs that echo, this book beckons you to step into a narrative that defies expectations.

This preface is an invitation to witness the drama, comedy, and romance of real-life stories, reminding you that in the labyrinth of intimate struggles, love is the guiding light. "Erect Cure" promises more than just insights; it's a promise of connection, understanding, and the uncharted heights of revitalized intimacy.

So, dear reader, fasten your seatbelt, for "Erect Cure" is not just a story; it's a thrilling expedition into the heart of human connection—a tale waiting to be discovered, experienced, and embraced with every beat of your heart.

CHAPTER ONE

Introduction to Erectile Dysfunction

In the hushed corridors of human intimacy, a silent struggle often unfolds—Erectile Dysfunction, a formidable adversary in the narrative of relationships. This clandestine antagonist, woven into the very fabric of human existence, manifests as a persistent inability to summon the physical ardor required for a dance as ancient as time itself.

Beneath the surface of shared moments and whispered promises, a complex interplay of physiological and psychological forces takes center stage. The symphony of nitric oxide, vascular dynamics, and hormonal intricacies orchestrates an intricate ballet, a delicate dance between pleasure and elusive performance.

Yet, as life weaves its intricate patterns, this delicate balance is often disrupted. Age, that inevitable sculptor of time, etches its marks on testosterone levels and vascular pathways.

Cardiovascular diseases emerge as silent architects, constructing barriers against the free flow of desire. Diabetes, a shadowy puppeteer, orchestrates nerve and vascular discord.

The narrative unfolds not only within the realms of the physical but takes a profound plunge into the ethereal landscapes of the mind. Stress, anxiety, and the ghostly specter of depression cast shadows on the stage, often eclipsing the spotlight that should illuminate the path to connection.

Smoking, a sorcerer of blood vessels, weaves spells of constriction, while alcohol and sedentary lifestyles contribute to the tapestry of challenges. Medications, with their dual roles as healers and disruptors, introduce unforeseen twists into the plot, altering the delicate equilibrium.

Diagnosis becomes a quest, a voyage through medical history and physical examinations, unraveling the intricate threads of causation. Laboratory tests paint a canvas of hormone levels and lipid profiles, while psychological assessments unveil the emotional hues that shape the narrative.

Amidst this intricate narrative, a diverse cast of treatments emerges. Medications, from the stalwart PDE5 inhibitors to the avant-garde alprostadil, offer pathways to rekindle the flame. Hormone therapy steps onto the stage, a silent maestro orchestrating hormonal harmony. Lifestyle changes, from the disciplined cadence of exercise to the symphony of a balanced diet, form the backdrop against which resilience takes center stage.

Yet, the plot extends beyond the physical, delving into the realm of the psyche. Counseling and therapy become pillars of support, guiding individuals and couples through the labyrinth of emotions. Relationships, caught in the ebb and flow, find solace in open communication and shared strategies for resilience.

As the narrative unfolds, the spotlight shifts to prevention, to the art of crafting a life that defies the clutches of this invisible adversary.

Healthy lifestyles emerge as protagonists, the guardians of a future untainted by the shadows of erectile challenges.

In the epilogue, the story transcends its immediate confines, extending into the realms of research and innovation. Stem cell therapy and shockwave therapy cast hopeful glimmers on the horizon, promising a future where the narrative of erectile resilience evolves into new chapters of triumph.

In this grand tapestry of human experience, Erectile Dysfunction emerges not as a singular antagonist but as a formidable challenge, met with resilience, understanding, and a collective quest for intimacy untethered by the shadows. The narrative persists, with each chapter unfolding a story of perseverance, connection, and the indomitable spirit to rise above.

Historical Context

The historical understanding of erectile dysfunction dates back centuries. In ancient times, various cultures had different beliefs about its causes, often attributing it to a mix of physical and spiritual factors. Ancient Greek and Roman writings mention treatments involving herbs, potions, and exercises.

During the Middle Ages, some medical texts proposed remedies like bloodletting and concoctions made from animal parts. In the Renaissance, anatomical knowledge improved, but misconceptions about sexuality persisted.

Well, we can confirm that it wasn't. As long as men have had penises (so, always), erectile dysfunction has been a hot topic, and doctors have been trying to combat it since time immemorial. The earliest recorded incidence of ED comes from India in the 8th century BC. The popular theory among doctors at the time was that ED was caused by having sex with "undesirable" women. Treatments included herbal medicines with additives from animals that were thought to increase desire or arousal. Alligators, mice, frogs, and sparrows were all animals that contributed to the concoctions of the time.

Fast forward several thousand years and, as an ED sufferer, you would have been introduced to the work of Dr. John R. Brinkley. The infamously fraudulent doctor dismissed (not unreasonably) the idea of using the extract of sheep testes to treat impotence, as had been the practice since the 1800s. Instead, Brinkley began promoting the use of transplanting goat testicles into men with ED, which was a very pricey and exclusive operation at the time. He was subsequently stripped of his bought medical licence, since such procedures were not regulated or approved at that period in time.

By the 1970s, penile implants had made a name for themselves as a solution for erectile dysfunction. At the same time, penile vacuum pumps were gaining popularity and Geddings Osbon's "youth equivalence device" (or YED) was paving the way for the penis vacuum devices that we are familiar with to this day.

The 1980s laid the groundwork for a sexual revolution with the research of Dr. Giles Brindley. Brindley injected a vasodilator into his veins, which caused corporal smooth muscle relaxation and induced an erection. His discovery led to research on vasodilators and alpha-blocking agents as a treatment for erectile dysfunction.

In the early 1990s, sildenafil was approved as a heart medication, and it was discovered that men taking the medication were experiencing firmer, longer-lasting erections. This led to further research on sildenafil as an erectile drug, and Pfizer unveiled Viagra in 1998. The drug exploded in popularity and now, nearly two decades later, it remains the most popular oral medication for erectile dysfunction.

In the 20th century, advancements in medicine led to a better understanding of the physiological aspects of erectile dysfunction. Psychological factors were also recognized as contributors. The development of medications like Viagra in the late 20th century revolutionized treatment.

Viagra has been extensively tested for safety and efficacy and continues to be the top contender in oral ED drugs. It is widely available with a prescription and also over the counter, and men now have the option to purchase Viagra online, making it even easier to get. The treatment of erectile dysfunction has come a long way from the days of potions and animal components and, for many men, life has never been better.

Prevalence and Demographics

Erectile dysfunction (ED) prevalence varies across different age groups and populations. Generally, it becomes more common with age. In men aged 40-70, the prevalence is estimated to be around 50%, with mild or moderate forms being more common than severe cases.

Factors such as diabetes, cardiovascular disease, obesity, and psychological issues can increase the risk of ED. Lifestyle factors like smoking and lack of physical activity are also linked.

Demographically, ED affects men of all races and ethnicities, but some studies suggest variations in prevalence among different groups. Additionally, cultural and socioeconomic factors can influence how individuals perceive and seek treatment for ED.

It's important to note that prevalence rates can change over time due to shifts in lifestyle, healthcare, and awareness. Seeking professional medical advice is crucial for accurate diagnosis and appropriate management of erectile dysfunction.

CHAPTER TWO

Physiological Basis of Erection

The male reproductive system is a complex network of organs designed for the production and delivery of sperm, as well as the secretion of hormones. At the core of this system is the pair of testes, which serve as the primary site for sperm production and also produce testosterone, a key male sex hormone.

Connected to the testes are the epididymis and vas deferens, which transport and store mature sperm. During ejaculation, sperm travel through the vas deferens and mix with fluids produced by the seminal vesicles and prostate gland. These fluids provide nourishment and help sperm move efficiently.

The penis, a crucial external organ, has three erectile chambers composed of spongy tissue. During arousal, these tissues fill with blood, causing the penis to become erect. The urethra, which runs through the penis, serves a dual purpose for both urine and semen transport.

Control of the male reproductive system involves a complex interplay of hormonal signals. The hypothalamus in the brain releases gonadotropin-releasing hormone (GnRH), stimulating the pituitary gland to release follicle-stimulating hormone (FSH) and luteinizing hormone (LH). These hormones, in turn, regulate the functions of the testes.

This intricate anatomy and physiology ensure the intricate processes of sperm production, transportation, and ejaculation, ultimately contributing to the male reproductive system's vital role in human reproduction.

Neurovascular mechanisms involved in achieving and maintaining an erection.

The achievement and maintenance of an erection involve intricate neurovascular mechanisms. The process is initiated by sexual arousal, which triggers a series of events:

1. Brain Stimulation:

Sexual thoughts or stimuli stimulate the brain, particularly the limbic system and hypothalamus. This activation leads to the release of neurotransmitters.

2. Release of Nitric Oxide (NO):

Sexual arousal prompts the release of nitric oxide from nerve endings and endothelial cells in the penis. Nitric oxide acts as a signaling molecule that relaxes smooth muscle cells within the erectile tissue.

3. Relaxation of Smooth Muscle:

Nitric oxide stimulates the production of cyclic guanosine monophosphate (cGMP), which, in turn, causes the smooth muscle cells in the erectile tissue to relax. This relaxation allows blood to flow into the penis, engorging the erectile chambers.

4. Increased Blood Flow:

As the smooth muscle relaxes, arterial blood flow to the penis increases. The corpora cavernosa, two erectile chambers in the penis, fill with blood, causing the penis to become erect.

5. Trapping of Blood:

The engorged erectile chambers compress the veins that usually allow blood to leave the penis. This compression helps trap blood within the penis, maintaining the erection.

6. Sustaining Erection:

The sustained erection is maintained by a delicate balance between factors that promote smooth muscle relaxation (like nitric oxide and cGMP) and those that counteract it. When sexual arousal diminishes, other enzymes break down cGMP, leading to the contraction of smooth muscle and decreased blood flow, allowing the penis to return to its flaccid state.

Disruptions in these neurovascular mechanisms, caused by factors like vascular issues, nerve damage, hormonal imbalances, or psychological factors, can contribute to erectile dysfunction. Understanding and addressing these factors are crucial for effective diagnosis and treatment.

Erectile dysfunction (ED) has a complex physiological basis involving both vascular and neurological components. Here's a brief overview:

1. Vascular Factors:

Blood Flow: Adequate blood flow to the penis is crucial for achieving and maintaining an erection. Conditions that affect blood vessels, such as atherosclerosis, can restrict blood flow, contributing to ED.

Endothelial Dysfunction: Dysfunction of the endothelium, the inner lining of blood vessels, can impact the ability of arteries to dilate properly, affecting blood flow to the penis.

2. Neurological Factors:

Nerve Signals: Nerve signals from the brain and spinal cord play a role in initiating and maintaining an erection. Conditions such as diabetes or spinal cord injuries can disrupt these signals.

Neurotransmitters: Chemicals like nitric oxide are released during sexual arousal, leading to the relaxation of smooth muscles in the penis. Disorders affecting neurotransmitter release can interfere with this process.

3. Hormonal Factors:

Testosterone Levels: While testosterone is a key hormone for sexual function, its role in ED is complex. Low testosterone levels alone might not be the sole cause of ED, but they can contribute, especially when combined with other factors.

4. Psychological Factors:

Mental Health: Anxiety, stress, depression, and relationship issues can contribute to or exacerbate ED. Psychological factors can interact with physiological aspects, creating a cycle of performance anxiety.

5. Medications and Lifestyle:

Certain medications, such as those for hypertension or depression, may have side effects impacting erectile function.

Lifestyle factors like smoking, excessive alcohol consumption, and lack of exercise can contribute to ED.

Understanding and addressing these physiological factors is crucial in diagnosing and treating erectile dysfunction. A comprehensive approach often involves lifestyle changes, psychological counseling, and, in some cases, medications or other medical interventions.

CHAPTER THREE

Causes and Risk Factors

Age-related factors.

As men age, there are several age-related factors and risk factors that can contribute to the development of erectile dysfunction (ED). Here are some key considerations:

1. Vascular Changes:

Aging can lead to changes in blood vessels, including atherosclerosis (hardening of the arteries), which may restrict blood flow to the penis, affecting erectile function.

2. Neurological Factors:

Nerve damage or deterioration over time can impact the transmission of signals between the brain and the penis, disrupting the neurovascular mechanisms involved in achieving and maintaining an erection.

3. Hormonal Changes:

Testosterone levels naturally decline with age. While lower testosterone alone may not cause ED, it can contribute, especially when combined with other factors.

4. Chronic Medical Conditions:

Conditions such as diabetes, hypertension, and cardiovascular diseases become more prevalent with age and are associated with an increased risk of ED.

5. Medications:

Certain medications commonly prescribed for age-related conditions, such as antihypertensives, antidepressants, and drugs for prostate issues, may have side effects that impact erectile function.

6. Psychological Factors:

Stress, anxiety, and depression, which may be more common in older individuals due to life changes and health concerns, can contribute to ED.

7. Lifestyle Factors:

Unhealthy lifestyle choices, such as smoking, excessive alcohol consumption, lack of physical activity, and poor diet, can contribute to vascular and overall health issues that may lead to ED.

Enlargement of the prostate (benign prostatic hyperplasia) or prostate cancer treatment can affect the structures surrounding the penis and impact erectile function.

While aging is a natural process, addressing modifiable risk factors through lifestyle changes, regular medical check-ups, and adopting a healthy approach to overall well-being can help mitigate the risk of developing age-related erectile dysfunction. Seeking medical advice is crucial for a comprehensive understanding of individual risk factors and appropriate management.

Cardiovascular Causes.

Cardiovascular issues are closely linked to erectile dysfunction (ED), and various cardiovascular peculiarities can contribute to the development of ED. Here are key implications:

1. Atherosclerosis:

Atherosclerosis, the hardening and narrowing of arteries, can affect blood flow to various parts of the body, including the penis. Reduced blood flow to the penile arteries is a common cause of ED.

2. Endothelial Dysfunction:

Cardiovascular diseases often lead to endothelial dysfunction, impairing the ability of blood vessels to dilate properly. In the context of ED, this dysfunction affects the blood vessels supplying the penis.

3. Hypertension (High Blood Pressure):

Hypertension is a known risk factor for ED. Elevated blood pressure can damage arteries, limiting blood flow to the penis and disrupting the neurovascular mechanisms involved in achieving and maintaining an erection.

4. Peripheral Arterial Disease (PAD):

PAD, a condition where narrowed arteries reduce blood flow to the extremities, including the penis, can contribute to ED.

5. Heart Disease:

Conditions such as coronary artery disease and heart failure are associated with an increased risk of ED. Shared risk factors, including vascular damage, contribute to this association.

6. Metabolic Syndrome:

Cardiovascular peculiarities associated with metabolic syndrome, such as insulin resistance and obesity, can indirectly contribute to ED through their impact on vascular and hormonal functions.

7. Medications:

Some medications prescribed for cardiovascular conditions, such as beta-blockers and diuretics, may have side effects that can affect erectile function.

8. Smoking:

Smoking is a major risk factor for both cardiovascular disease and ED. It damages blood vessels and can exacerbate existing cardiovascular issues, contributing to ED.

Dyslipidemia, or abnormal levels of lipids in the blood, is associated with cardiovascular disease and may contribute to ED.

Addressing cardiovascular health through lifestyle changes, such as maintaining a healthy diet, regular exercise, and managing risk factors like hypertension and high cholesterol, is essential for preventing or managing ED associated with cardiovascular peculiarities. Seeking guidance from healthcare professionals is crucial for a comprehensive approach to both cardiovascular health and sexual well-being.

Diabetes and metabolic syndrome.

Diabetes and metabolic syndrome can significantly contribute to the development of erectile dysfunction (ED) through various physiological mechanisms. Here are key implications:

1. Vascular Damage:

Diabetes and metabolic syndrome often lead to vascular complications. Elevated blood sugar levels can damage blood vessels, including those supplying the penis. This vascular damage restricts blood flow, a crucial factor in achieving and maintaining an erection.

2. Nerve Damage (Neuropathy):

Prolonged high blood sugar levels can cause nerve damage (neuropathy). Nerves play a crucial role in transmitting signals between the brain and the penis, and any disruption in this communication can lead to difficulties in achieving or sustaining an erection.

3. Endothelial Dysfunction:

Diabetes and metabolic syndrome can result in endothelial dysfunction, affecting the inner lining of blood vessels. This dysfunction contributes to impaired relaxation of the smooth muscles in the penile arteries, further compromising blood flow.

4. Hormonal Imbalances:

Insulin resistance, a common feature of metabolic syndrome, can lead to hormonal imbalances. Changes in insulin levels may affect testosterone production, contributing to erectile dysfunction.

5. Inflammation:

Chronic inflammation, common in metabolic syndrome, can contribute to ED. Inflammation may affect the endothelial cells and smooth muscle tissue in the penis, disrupting normal erectile function.

6. Obesity:

Metabolic syndrome is often associated with obesity. Excess body fat, especially around the abdomen, is linked to increased insulin resistance and inflammation, both of which contribute to the risk of ED.

7. Medications:

Some medications commonly prescribed for diabetes or related conditions may have side effects that impact erectile function.

8. Psychological Impact:

Coping with chronic diseases like diabetes and managing lifestyle changes can lead to stress, anxiety, and depression, which are additional psychological factors that can contribute to ED.

Managing diabetes and metabolic syndrome through lifestyle modifications, medication adherence, and regular medical check-ups is crucial in mitigating the risk of erectile dysfunction. Seeking guidance from healthcare professionals helps tailor a comprehensive approach to address both the underlying conditions and their potential impact on sexual health.

CHAPTER FOUR

Psychological Factors of Erectile Dysfunction

Stress and anxiety.

Psychological factors, particularly stress and anxiety, play a significant role in erectile dysfunction (ED). Here are key aspects of their impact:

1. Performance Anxiety:

The fear of not performing well sexually, known as performance anxiety, can create a cycle of stress and ED. Anxiety about one's sexual performance may lead to heightened stress, making it difficult to achieve or maintain an erection.

2. General Anxiety and Stress:

Chronic stress and anxiety, whether related to work, relationships, or other life challenges, can contribute to ED. The body's stress response involves the release of hormones like cortisol, which, when elevated over time, can negatively affect sexual function.

Stress and anxiety can alter the balance of neurotransmitters in the brain, affecting the signals involved in sexual arousal and response. This disruption can contribute to difficulties in achieving or sustaining an erection.

High levels of cortisol, a stress hormone, may impair the production of nitric oxide, a key component in the neurovascular mechanisms leading to erections. Reduced nitric oxide availability can hinder blood flow to the penis.

Depression often coexists with anxiety and stress, and it is another psychological factor linked to ED. Feelings of sadness, hopelessness, and low self-esteem can contribute to sexual difficulties.

Relationship stress or conflicts can contribute to ED. Communication issues, emotional distance, or unresolved conflicts between partners may impact sexual intimacy.

Persistent negative thoughts related to sexual performance can create a self-fulfilling prophecy. These thoughts can increase anxiety and stress, further exacerbating ED.

Psychological factors can interfere with the effectiveness of physical treatments for ED. Even if there is a physical cause, the presence of anxiety or stress can worsen the condition.

Addressing the psychological aspects of ED often involves a combination of therapies, including cognitive-behavioral therapy (CBT), counseling, and stress management techniques. Open communication with a healthcare professional can help identify and address these factors, leading to a more holistic approach to managing erectile dysfunction.

CHAPTER FIVE

Lifestyle Factors of Erectile Dysfunction

The link between lifestyle factors, including alcohol consumption, obesity, and smoking, and erectile dysfunction (ED) is well-established and multifaceted.

Alcohol Consumption:

Excessive alcohol consumption is associated with both acute and chronic effects on sexual function. In the short term, alcohol acts as a depressant on the central nervous system, potentially impairing sexual performance. Long-term alcohol abuse can lead to liver damage, hormonal imbalances, and cardiovascular issues, all of which contribute to ED. Additionally, alcohol can decrease testosterone levels, disrupt the neurovascular mechanisms involved in erections, and contribute to psychological factors such as anxiety and depression.

Obesity is a significant risk factor for ED. Excess body weight, particularly abdominal obesity, is associated with insulin resistance, inflammation, and dyslipidemia. These metabolic abnormalities contribute to vascular damage and endothelial dysfunction, limiting blood flow to the penis. Obesity is also linked to hormonal imbalances, including reduced testosterone levels, which play a role in erectile function. Furthermore, obesity can contribute to psychological factors such as body image issues and low self-esteem, which may exacerbate ED.

Smoking is a well-established risk factor for ED. Tobacco smoke contains numerous harmful substances that contribute to vascular damage, reducing blood flow to the penis. Nicotine, a vasoconstrictor, narrows blood vessels, further compromising erectile function. Smoking is associated with a higher risk of atherosclerosis, which can impact the arteries supplying the genitals. Additionally, smoking is linked to oxidative stress and inflammation, both of which contribute to overall vascular health and may affect erectile function.

Interplay of Lifestyle Factors:

It's important to note that these lifestyle factors often interact, amplifying their impact on ED. For instance, smoking and excessive alcohol consumption often coexist with poor dietary choices and sedentary behavior, contributing to obesity and compounding the risk of ED. Moreover, the psychological stress associated with these lifestyle factors can exacerbate the condition, creating a cycle of worsening erectile function.

Addressing Lifestyle Factors:

Addressing lifestyle factors is a crucial component of ED management. Lifestyle modifications, including reducing alcohol consumption, achieving and maintaining a healthy weight, quitting smoking, and adopting a balanced diet, can significantly improve vascular health and overall well-being, thereby mitigating the risk and severity of ED. Seeking professional guidance for a personalized approach to lifestyle changes is advisable for individuals experiencing erectile dysfunction.

CHAPTER SIX

Medical Conditions and Medications Contributing to Erectile Dysfunction

Medical Conditions

1. Cardiovascular Diseases:

Atherosclerosis, hypertension, coronary artery disease, and peripheral arterial disease can impede blood flow to the penis, contributing to erectile dysfunction.

2. Diabetes:

Diabetes can lead to nerve damage (neuropathy) and vascular issues, both of which are significant contributors to erectile dysfunction.

3. Neurological Disorders:

Conditions such as multiple sclerosis, Parkinson's disease, and spinal cord injuries can disrupt nerve signals involved in sexual function.

4. Hormonal Imbalances:

Low testosterone levels, often associated with conditions like hypogonadism, can contribute to erectile dysfunction.

5. Endocrine Disorders:

Disorders affecting the endocrine system, including thyroid disorders and adrenal gland abnormalities, may impact hormonal balance and erectile function.

6. Pelvic Surgery and Radiation:

Surgical procedures or radiation therapy in the pelvic area, especially for prostate cancer, can damage nerves and blood vessels critical for erections.

7. Peyronie's Disease:

Peyronie's disease involves the development of fibrous scar tissue within the penis, causing curvature and potentially leading to erectile dysfunction.

8. Chronic Kidney Disease:

Kidney disease can contribute to endothelial dysfunction and hormonal imbalances, impacting erectile function.

9. Liver Cirrhosis:

Advanced liver disease, such as cirrhosis, can lead to hormonal imbalances and vascular issues that affect sexual health.

10. Chronic Obstructive Pulmonary Disease (COPD):

Respiratory conditions like COPD may impact oxygen levels in the blood, affecting overall vascular health and potentially leading to erectile dysfunction.

11. Medication Side Effects:

Certain medications, including those for hypertension, antidepressants, and some prostate-related drugs, can have side effects that contribute to ED.

12. Psychological Conditions:

Anxiety, depression, and chronic stress can significantly impact sexual function, leading to or exacerbating erectile dysfunction.

13. Obesity:

Excess body weight, particularly abdominal obesity, is associated with metabolic and vascular issues that contribute to erectile dysfunction.

Conditions like sleep apnea can contribute to hormonal imbalances and affect overall health, potentially influencing erectile function.

Autoimmune conditions, such as rheumatoid arthritis or lupus, can contribute to systemic inflammation that may impact erectile function.

Understanding the connection between these medical conditions and erectile dysfunction is crucial for accurate diagnosis and appropriate management. Individuals experiencing persistent or worsening symptoms should seek guidance from healthcare professionals for a comprehensive assessment and personalized treatment plan.

Side effects of Medications

1. Antihypertensive Medications:

Beta-Blockers: Certain beta-blockers, such as propranolol and metoprolol, are associated with erectile dysfunction.

2. Antidepressants:

Selective Serotonin Reuptake Inhibitors **(SSRIs)**: Medications like fluoxetine, sertraline, and paroxetine are known to have sexual side effects, including ED.

Tricyclic Antidepressants: Amitriptyline and imipramine are examples of tricyclic antidepressants that may contribute to erectile dysfunction.

3. Antipsychotics:

Risperidone: This antipsychotic medication has been associated with sexual side effects, including ED.

4. Anti-Anxiety Medications:

Benzodiazepines: Some benzodiazepines, like diazepam and lorazepam, may have sexual side effects, although the evidence is not as strong as with other drug classes.

5. Hormonal Medications:

5-alpha Reductase Inhibitors: Medications like finasteride and dutasteride, used for benign prostatic hyperplasia (BPH) and male pattern baldness, may have sexual side effects, including ED.

6. Chemotherapy Drugs:

Cisplatin: Some chemotherapy drugs, including cisplatin, may have adverse effects on sexual function.

7. Antiarrhythmics:

Amiodarone: This antiarrhythmic medication has been associated with sexual side effects, including erectile dysfunction.

8. Hormonal Contraceptives:

Progestin-Only Contraceptives: Some progestin-only contraceptives, such as certain birth control pills and injections, may have an impact on sexual function.

9. Gastric Acid Suppressants:

H2 Blockers: Medications like cimetidine, used to reduce stomach acid, have been linked to sexual side effects, including ED.

Baclofen: This muscle relaxant may have sexual side effects, although the evidence is limited.

It's important to note that not everyone will experience sexual side effects from these medications, and individual responses can vary. If someone is concerned about the impact of a specific medication on sexual function, it's advisable to consult with a healthcare professional. They can provide guidance on potential alternatives or adjustments to the treatment plan while considering the overall health and well-being of the individual.

CHAPTER SEVEN

Diagnosis and Assessment of Erectile Dysfunction

Medical history and physical examination.

Below is a sample, but non-exhausive. It is to enable one better prepare for Hospital Appointments

Medical History:

Mr. X, a 55-year-old male, presented with concerns about erectile dysfunction (ED). Gathering a comprehensive medical history is crucial in understanding potential contributing factors:

Chief Complaint: Mr. Smith reports difficulty achieving and maintaining an erection sufficient for sexual intercourse over the past six months.

Onset and Duration: Inquire about the gradual onset or sudden occurrence of symptoms, as well as the duration and progression of ED.

Frequency and Severity: Explore the frequency and severity of erectile difficulties. Does it occur consistently or intermittently? Is there a specific trigger or pattern?

Associated Symptoms: Ask about other associated symptoms, such as decreased libido, premature ejaculation, or pain during intercourse.

Medical History: Assess for underlying medical conditions, such as diabetes, cardiovascular disease, hypertension, or neurological disorders, which may contribute to ED.

Medication History: Review current and past medications, as certain drugs like antihypertensives, antidepressants, and hormonal treatments may have ED as a side effect.

Psychosocial Factors: Inquire about stressors, anxiety, or relationship issues that might impact sexual function. Assess for symptoms of depression or other psychological conditions.

Lifestyle Factors: Explore lifestyle habits, including smoking, alcohol consumption, and exercise, as these can influence erectile function.

Conducting a thorough physical examination helps identify potential physical causes of ED. It is advisable to allow only your Health Care provider do this assessment so as t get a unique and workable diagnosis for you or your loved one.

Blood Pressure Measurement: Assess blood pressure to identify hypertension, a common risk factor for ED.

Body Mass Index (BMI): Calculate BMI to evaluate for obesity, which is associated with metabolic and vascular issues contributing to ED.

Genital Examination: Examine the genitals for signs of Peyronie's disease, abnormalities, or structural issues that may impact erectile function.

Neurological Examination: Conduct a neurological examination to assess for abnormalities that could affect nerve function, such as reflexes and sensation in the genital area.

Cardiovascular Examination: Perform a cardiovascular examination to identify potential signs of atherosclerosis or other vascular issues affecting blood flow.

Testicular Examination: Examine the testicles for any abnormalities that might indicate an underlying condition impacting testosterone production.

Digital Rectal Examination (DRE): For men over 40, consider a DRE to assess the prostate, especially if there are concerns about prostate-related issues.

Collaborating with the patient to gather this detailed medical history and perform a comprehensive physical examination provides a foundation for understanding the potential causes of ED and guiding further diagnostic and treatment options. Referral to a specialist may be warranted for more in-depth evaluations, such as vascular studies or hormonal assessments.

Diagnostic tests and tools.

Several diagnostic tools and tests can be utilized to assess and diagnose erectile dysfunction (ED). The choice of tests often depends on the individual's medical history, physical examination findings, and suspected underlying causes. Here are some commonly used diagnostic tools for ED:

1. Medical History:

A detailed medical history, including information about the onset, duration, and progression of ED, as well as any associated symptoms, can provide valuable insights.

2. Sexual Health Questionnaires:

Specific questionnaires, such as the International Index of Erectile Function (IIEF), may be used to quantify the severity of erectile dysfunction and its impact on sexual function.

3. Blood Tests:

Hormone Levels: Measurement of testosterone and other relevant hormones to assess hormonal imbalances.

Blood Glucose Levels: Particularly important in individuals with diabetes.

Lipid Profile: To evaluate for dyslipidemia, which is associated with vascular issues.

4. Penile Doppler Ultrasound:

This test assesses blood flow to the penis by using ultrasound to measure the velocity of blood in the penile arteries. It can help identify vascular issues.

5. Nocturnal Penile Tumescence (NPT) Test:

NPT monitoring involves placing a device around the penis to measure nocturnal erections. It helps determine whether the ED is primarily psychological or has a physical basis.

6. Injection Test (Penile Injection Test):

A pharmacological agent, such as alprostadil, is injected directly into the penis to induce an erection. This test helps assess the vascular and smooth muscle function of the penis.

7. Cavernosometry and Cavernosography:

These tests involve injecting a contrast agent into the penile vasculature and using imaging techniques to evaluate blood flow and detect any structural abnormalities.

8. Dynamic Infusion Cavernosometry (DICC):

This test measures penile blood pressure and flow during an erection induced by injecting a vasoactive substance into the penis.

9. Psychological Evaluation:

For individuals with suspected psychological causes, a psychological evaluation or consultation with a mental health professional may be recommended.

10. Pelvic and Abdominal Imaging:

Imaging studies, such as pelvic or abdominal scans, may be conducted to identify structural issues affecting the reproductive organs.

11. Peyronie's Disease Assessment:

Evaluation for Peyronie's disease may include imaging studies, such as ultrasound or magnetic resonance imaging (MRI), to assess penile curvature and fibrotic plaques.

It's essential to note that the choice of diagnostic tools depends on the individual case, and healthcare professionals may use a combination of these tests for a thorough assessment. A collaborative approach between the patient and healthcare provider is crucial for accurate diagnosis and effective treatment planning for erectile dysfunction.

CHAPTER EIGHT

Treatment Options

Treatment options for erectile dysfunction (ED) vary depending on the underlying causes and individual health factors. Here are common approaches:

1. Lifestyle Modifications:

Healthy Diet and Exercise: Adopting a healthy diet and engaging in regular physical activity can improve overall cardiovascular health, addressing one of the common causes of ED.

Weight Management: Maintaining a healthy weight can positively impact hormonal balance and vascular health.

2. Psychotherapy:

Counseling and Sex Therapy: Addressing psychological factors contributing to ED, such as anxiety or relationship issues, through counseling or sex therapy can be beneficial.

Phosphodiesterase Type 5 (PDE5) Inhibitors: Drugs like sildenafil (Viagra), tadalafil (Cialis), vardenafil (Levitra), and avanafil are commonly prescribed. They enhance the effects of nitric oxide, promoting blood flow to the penis.

Alprostadil: Injected directly into the penis, alprostadil dilates blood vessels and increases blood flow, aiding in achieving an erection.

Alprostadil Suppositories: Inserted into the urethra, these suppositories also promote blood flow to the penis.

6. Vacuum Erection Devices (VEDs):

Mechanical devices create a vacuum, drawing blood into the penis and facilitating an erection. A constriction ring is then placed at the base to maintain the erection.

7. Penile Implants:

Surgical implants, such as inflatable or malleable prostheses, are implanted into the penis to provide rigidity when desired.

8. Hormone Replacement Therapy (HRT):

Testosterone Replacement: In cases of low testosterone levels, hormone replacement therapy may be considered.

9. Shockwave Therapy:

Low-intensity shockwaves are applied to the penis to stimulate new blood vessel formation and enhance blood flow. This is a relatively new treatment option.

Strengthening pelvic floor muscles may improve erectile function, especially if ED is related to muscle weakness.

Some individuals explore acupuncture as an alternative therapy to improve blood flow and address underlying imbalances.

It's crucial for individuals experiencing ED to consult with a healthcare professional to determine the most suitable treatment approach based on their specific condition and health history. Combining treatments or addressing multiple factors simultaneously may be necessary for optimal results.

CHAPTER NINE

Emerging Therapies and Researches

Emerging therapies and ongoing research in erectile dysfunction (ED) aim to provide novel treatment options and deepen our understanding of the condition. Several exciting developments and potential therapies are being explored:

1. Stem Cell Therapy:

Stem cell therapy holds promise in regenerating damaged tissues and improving blood vessel function in the penis. Early studies suggest the potential for enhanced erectile function with this innovative approach.

2. Platelet-Rich Plasma (PRP):

PRP involves injecting a concentrated form of the patient's own platelets into the penis. This therapy aims to stimulate tissue repair and regeneration, potentially improving erectile function.

3. Gene Therapy:

Gene therapy is being investigated to target specific genetic factors contributing to ED. This approach seeks to introduce or modify genes to address underlying causes and improve overall penile health.

4. Nitrates and Nitric Oxide Donors:

Research continues on medications that release nitric oxide or mimic its effects, aiming to enhance the natural mechanisms involved in achieving and maintaining an erection.

5. Melanocortin Receptor Agonists:

Melanocortin receptor agonists are being explored for their potential in promoting erections. These drugs influence neural pathways involved in sexual arousal and may offer an alternative treatment option.

6. Phosphodiesterase Type 5 (PDE5) Inhibitors:

While PDE5 inhibitors like Viagra have been effective, ongoing research seeks to develop next-generation PDE5 inhibitors with improved efficacy and fewer side effects.

7. Novel Delivery Methods:

Researchers are exploring alternative delivery methods for existing medications, such as topical gels or patches, to enhance convenience and reduce potential side effects.

8. Cannabinoids:

Some studies are investigating the role of cannabinoids, particularly cannabidiol (CBD), in improving erectile function. The complex interaction between the endocannabinoid system and sexual health is an area of growing interest.

9. MicroRNA Therapies:

MicroRNAs are small RNA molecules that regulate gene expression. Researchers are studying their potential role in modulating pathways related to erectile function and exploring microRNA-based therapies.

Techniques involving electrical stimulation or neuromodulation are being investigated to influence nerve pathways and enhance penile blood flow, potentially providing new avenues for treatment.

While these emerging therapies show promise, it's essential to approach them with caution until further research confirms their safety and effectiveness. As the field of ED research advances, the hope is to offer a wider range of targeted and personalized treatment options for individuals experiencing erectile dysfunction.

CHAPTER TEN

Impact of Relationships

Erectile dysfunction (ED) can have a profound impact on relationships, extending beyond its physical implications to affect emotional intimacy and overall relationship dynamics. The consequences of ED often extend to both partners, shaping their experiences and interactions in various ways.

1. Communication Challenges:

ED can create communication challenges between partners. The affected individual may struggle to express their feelings, fearing judgment or a sense of inadequacy. Partners may also find it difficult to broach the topic sensitively, potentially leading to misunderstandings.

2. Emotional Strain:

The emotional toll of ED can be significant. Individuals experiencing ED may grapple with feelings of frustration, embarrassment, and diminished self-esteem. Partners may experience concern, empathy, or frustration, navigating their own emotional responses to the situation.

3. Diminished Intimacy:

ED often results in a decline in sexual intimacy, impacting the overall connection between partners. The absence of regular sexual activity may lead to a sense of emotional distance, affecting the quality of the relationship.

4. Self-Esteem Issues:

Individuals with ED may face challenges related to self-esteem and self-worth. The perceived inability to meet societal or personal expectations of masculinity can contribute to feelings of inadequacy.

5. Relationship Stress:

The stress associated with ED can spill over into other aspects of the relationship. Ongoing concerns about sexual performance may create an atmosphere of tension and strain, potentially leading to conflicts in other areas of the relationship.

6. Changes in Relationship Dynamics:

Partners may witness shifts in relationship dynamics, as the focus on sexual performance may overshadow other aspects of the relationship. The couple may need to navigate these changes and work towards maintaining a balanced and supportive connection.

8. Seeking Professional Help:

Couples may choose to seek professional guidance, such as sex therapy or couples counseling, to address the emotional and relational challenges posed by ED. Professional support can offer a safe space for both partners to express their concerns and work towards solutions.

While ED can present challenges, it is crucial for couples to recognize that it is a medical condition with various treatment options. By approaching the issue as a shared challenge and fostering open communication, couples can strengthen their bond, demonstrating resilience and mutual support in the face of adversity.

Strategies for coping and support.

Couples often need to develop coping strategies together. Open communication, empathy, and a willingness to explore alternative forms of intimacy become essential components in managing the emotional impact of ED.. Here are some coping strategies for couples:

1. Open Communication:

Foster a safe and open environment for discussing feelings, concerns, and expectations related to ED. Clear communication helps both partners understand each other's perspectives.

2. Educate Yourselves:

Learn about erectile dysfunction together. Understanding the physical and psychological factors involved can demystify the condition and reduce feelings of blame or inadequacy.

3. Seek Professional Guidance:

Consider couples counseling or sex therapy. A qualified professional can provide a supportive space for both partners to express their emotions, work through challenges, and explore strategies for coping with ED.

4. Explore Alternative Intimacy:

Embrace non-sexual forms of intimacy. Focus on emotional connection, affectionate touch, and shared activities that strengthen the bond between partners.

5. Encourage Healthful Habits:

Support each other in adopting a healthy lifestyle. Engage in regular exercise, maintain a balanced diet, and manage stress together, as these factors can positively impact overall health, including sexual function.

6. Participate in Treatment Decisions:

If the individual with ED seeks medical treatment, involve both partners in the decision-making process. Discuss potential treatments, address concerns, and attend medical appointments together for mutual understanding.

7. Manage Expectations:

Adjust expectations regarding sexual performance. Recognize that intimacy can take various forms, and a focus on emotional connection can enhance the overall relationship.

8. Encourage Professional Support for the Individual with ED:

Support and encourage the individual with ED to seek medical advice and treatment. Accompanying them to medical appointments and actively participating in the treatment plan can strengthen the sense of partnership.

9. Maintain a Positive Atmosphere:

Cultivate a positive and understanding atmosphere within the relationship. Focus on shared joys and achievements, reinforcing the notion that ED is just one aspect of the relationship.

10. Stay Patient and Supportive:

Patience is crucial. Support each other through the ups and downs of managing ED. Recognize that progress may take time, and celebrate small victories together.

11. Explore Mutual Hobbies and Activities:

Engaging in activities that both partners enjoy can create shared positive experiences, fostering a sense of connection outside of the context of ED.

Intimacy coaching or attending intimacy workshops together can provide additional tools and techniques for enhancing emotional and physical connection.

By approaching ED as a shared challenge and working together to find solutions, couples can strengthen their relationship and build resilience. The key is to maintain open communication, offer mutual support, and explore new ways to connect intimately beyond traditional expectations.

CHAPTER ELEVEN

Prevention and Healthy Lifestyle Habits

While not all cases of erectile dysfunction (ED) can be prevented, adopting a healthy lifestyle and addressing potential risk factors may contribute to maintaining erectile function. Here are strategies to help prevent or reduce the risk of developing ED:

1. Maintain a Healthy Lifestyle:

Adopt a balanced diet rich in fruits, vegetables, whole grains, and lean proteins. Limit saturated fats and sugars, which can contribute to cardiovascular issues.

2. Regular Exercise:

Engage in regular physical activity. Exercise improves overall cardiovascular health, which is crucial for adequate blood flow to the penis.

3. Maintain a Healthy Weight:

Obesity is a risk factor for ED. Achieving and maintaining a healthy weight through diet and exercise can positively impact erectile function.

4. Manage Chronic Conditions:

Control chronic conditions such as diabetes and hypertension through medication, lifestyle modifications, and regular medical check-ups.

5. Quit Smoking:

Smoking damages blood vessels and restricts blood flow, increasing the risk of ED. Quitting smoking is a significant step in preventing or mitigating erectile dysfunction.

6. Limit Alcohol Consumption:

Excessive alcohol consumption can contribute to ED. Moderating alcohol intake, especially for those at risk, is advisable.

7. Manage Stress:

Chronic stress can contribute to ED. Incorporate stress-reducing techniques such as meditation, deep breathing exercises, or yoga into daily life.

8. Prioritize Mental Health:

Address and manage psychological factors such as anxiety and depression. Seeking counseling or therapy can be beneficial.

9. Regular Check-ups:

Schedule regular medical check-ups to monitor overall health and address any emerging health issues promptly.

10. Avoid Illicit Drug Use:

Illicit drugs, especially those that impact the cardiovascular system, can contribute to ED. Avoiding drug use is essential for maintaining sexual health.

11. Get Adequate Sleep:

Quality sleep is crucial for overall health, including hormonal balance. Aim for 7-9 hours of sleep per night.

12. Practice Safe Sex:

Protecting oneself from sexually transmitted infections (STIs) is vital. STIs can contribute to conditions that may lead to ED.

13. Limit Bicycle Riding Time:

Prolonged pressure on the perineum during cycling may contribute to ED. Using a proper bike seat and taking breaks during long rides can help prevent this.

14. Stay Hydrated:

Proper hydration supports overall health, including cardiovascular health, and can contribute to erectile function.

15. Limit Caffeine Intake:

Excessive caffeine intake may contribute to anxiety and interfere with sleep, impacting overall health and potentially affecting erectile function.

While these strategies can contribute to overall health and may reduce the risk of developing ED, it's important to remember that individual factors vary. If concerns about erectile function arise, seeking prompt medical advice is crucial for accurate diagnosis and appropriate management.

CHAPTER TWELVE

Erectile Dysfunction – My Story

- Mr. Bruce

My name is Bruce. I was a public servant for 27 years. When I was in my late forties, I set up a gardening business in a bid to marry my interest in golf with horticulture. Despite my best efforts, I never did get a job as a groundsman on a golf course but the business ran for several years regardless. Now I'm 71 and retired. Soon I'll be celebrating 50 years of marriage.

When I was 57, I was diagnosed with erectile dysfunction (ED), which is an inability to get or keep an erection during sexual intercourse. While I'm really comfortable talking about this issue now, I'd never discussed it with any other guys. I guess no one wants to admit to it.

My sex life had been a disaster for several years. I was having 'improper' erections that weren't firm. I would ejaculate about a minute into intercourse. This was no good for my wife, and no good for me. I felt like I wasn't performing, that I was failing her. She thought I no longer found her attractive. But it didn't have anything to do with her at all.

I'd heard about Viagra on the grapevine and decided to go to my doctor to ask about it.

It was very clear to the GP from the outset that my problem was caused by smoking, which can affect your circulation, including your circulation down there. I had no idea of the link between erectile dysfunction and smoking but he made the connection straight away. If I'd known, I would have gone much earlier.

I've since spoken with friends with ED who are younger than me. One had his prostate removed for cancer. The surgery for this often cuts some nerves which causes ED. ED can also be a side effect of some drugs for high blood pressure. The reasons for the problem can be different for different blokes.

In my case, I'd been smoking for 37 years. I'd never considered giving up before because I thought I was too addicted. But once I made the connection, I said to myself that if I'm going to fix this problem, the smoking's got to go.

My GP put me onto a drug called Zyban which is acts like a mind bending drug that gets you to a stage where you don't want to have cigarettes. It can have some side-effects so it's not for everyone. In my case it worked – I gave up smoking within seven days.

At the same time, my GP put me on Viagra. This worked very well, with minimal side effects. When on it, some people can get a bit of a headache, or feel a little flushed. After a time, I tried other drugs for erectile dysfunction called Cialis and Levitra. All three worked well, but after some years, they began not to work at all.

When I went back to my GP to see what my options were, he referred me to a urologist. When I met with the urologist about my problem, he said he had seen a lot of blokes from my golf club for the exact same issue! It made me realise how common it is.

I asked about other treatments I'd researched on the internet, like a pellet that you put into the tip of the penis. He said that was ''old hat, like putting soap in there''.

He recommended I try intracavernosal injections. They involve horizontally injecting a compound drug with a very fine needle into the base of the penis. I thought it was worth giving a go.

A nurse demonstrated the procedure in the specialist's rooms the first time. It didn't hurt. Once you're shown how to do it, you do it yourself at home. There are some helpful videos online. You inject prior to intercourse and the effects last for about four hours. I've been successfully doing it for three years now and haven't experienced any side effects.

What I would say to other men is that if you are having the same problem, the first step is to go and speak to your GP to get the ball rolling. This isn't something to be scared of. While I was initially a bit embarrassed, doing something about it has been worth it. It's restored my confidence and really helped my relationship. I only wish I'd done it earlier.

- Anonymous

I am 38-years-old and have been with my partner for almost four years. I have had Type 2 diabetes for five years and use insulin five times a day.

"Over the last three and a half years I've suffered from severe neuropathy, so I'm on medication for that and also take tablets to lower my blood pressure.

I first noticed my erection problems about two years ago. The desire was still strong, but when it came to the point of penetration, my erection simply vanished. In the past, I have never had any problems getting and maintaining an erection so it came as quite a surprise.

"My partner and I have always enjoyed a loving and active sex life. At first I questioned our relationship. Did I still find her attractive? Was I looking at other women? Had the relationship changed in some way? Through sheer process of elimination, I came to realise the problem was mechanical.

"During this period, it affected our sexual relationship up to a point, but not in a detrimental way. Even though I wasn't always able to perform penetrative sex, she was quite happy to be stimulated in other ways.

"Luckily, my partner and I talk freely about everything and we were able to discuss the problem without too many inhibitions. I reassured her it was nothing to do with her and that I thought it was linked to my diabetes.

"I have a light-hearted relationship with my diabetes team so I didn't have a problem speaking to them about it.

"The next time I was due for a doctor's appointment, I told my GP about the erectile problems. She was very helpful and gave me a list of the drugs available and I opted for Cialis.

"It didn't take long to get used to the tablets. I take one about half an hour before I think we might have sex. More than 50 per cent of the time I can do without the tablets, but it's good to know they are there as a back up. One tablet lasts for about 36 hours.

"My partner was very happy to give the tablets a go. She prefers me to try without the tablets, but she has no real problem with them.

"I haven't suffered any side effects and although it slightly takes the spontaneity away, our sex life is as active and healthy as ever."

CONCLUSION

In the closing pages of "Erect Cure," we find not just an end but a beginning—a journey that transcends the realm of erectile dysfunction and embraces the Penile of revitalized intimacy. As we bid farewell to the challenges explored within these chapters, remember that each obstacle faced was a stepping stone toward a summit of rekindled connection.

In the ascent from the depths of uncertainty, we've uncovered tales of resilience, courage, and the transformative power of understanding. "Erect Cure" isn't just a book; it's an invitation to rise above the shadows of ED, reaching for the pinnacle of shared joy and fulfillment.

Amidst the celebration of triumphs, let us not forget a humble yet vital reminder—your journey doesn't end here. As the last page turns, may it be a gentle prompt to seek the guidance of healthcare professionals. Their expertise can illuminate personalized paths, ensuring that your pursuit of intimacy continues to ascend.

May this narrative linger in your thoughts as a beacon of hope, reminding you that the Penile

isn't merely a destination but a state of being—
one where love and intimacy flourish. Here's to
the Penile, the lift, and the everlasting journey
toward a love that knows no boundaries.

ACKNOWLEDGMENT

In the tapestry of "Erect Cure," the threads of gratitude weave through the heartfelt stories and shared experiences of those who have generously contributed to this exploration of intimate challenges and triumphs.

To the individuals and their partners who opened their hearts, bared their souls, and allowed their narratives to become the essence of this book, your courage and vulnerability have shaped its very core.

A special acknowledgment to the healthcare professionals whose expertise and compassionate care illuminate the path toward restored intimacy. Your dedication to the well-being of others is a beacon of hope in the realm of erectile dysfunction.

To Ms. Elizabeth Cyril who gave enormous secretarial assistance in the typing and formatting of the manuscript.

To the friends, family, and allies who provided unwavering support throughout this literary endeavor, your encouragement has been a source of inspiration and strength.

This work is a collaborative creation, and I extend profound appreciation to everyone who played a role, no matter how small, in bringing "Erect Cure" to life. May this book be a testament to the power of shared stories, empathetic understanding, and the infinite possibilities that arise when love becomes the guiding force.

With heartfelt gratitude,

. . .

Dr. Harry Chew

Disclaimer:

This book provides information and guidance intended for general educational purposes only. It is not a substitute for professional medical advice, diagnosis, or treatment. Readers should consult with a qualified healthcare professional for personalized recommendations regarding their specific condition. The author and publisher disclaim any liability arising directly or indirectly from the use of the information provided in this book. Individual responses to exercises, treatments, or lifestyle changes may vary, and readers should exercise caution and seek medical guidance before implementing any suggestions contained herein.

www.ingramcontent.com/pod-product-compliance
Lightning Source LLC
Chambersburg PA
CBHW070750250726

48662CB00004B/1725